Table Of Contents

Chapter 1: Introduction to Farm-to-Table Dining

The Farm-to-Table Movement Explained

A burgeoning culinary movement known as "Farm-to-Table" places a focus on obtaining products directly from local producers and growers. As people's awareness of the origins of their food and its effects on the environment has grown in recent years, so has the popularity of this movement.

Restaurant owners who embrace the Farm-to-Table philosophy are committed to using fresh, seasonal ingredients that are grown or raised in a sustainable and ethical manner. By working closely with local farmers and producers, these restaurant owners are able to create dishes that are not only delicious but also support the local economy and promote environmental sustainability.

For parents and adults looking to lead a healthier lifestyle, the Farm-to-Table movement offers a way to enjoy fresh, organic and chemical-free produce that is free from harmful pesticides and chemicals induce fertiliser. By choosing farm-fresh ingredients, families can ensure that they are getting the highest quality food that is packed with nutrients and mouth watering flavour.

For those following specific diets such as vegan, gluten-free, or Paleo, the Farm-to-Table movement provides a wide range of options to suit their needs. By using locally sourced ingredients, restaurants can easily accommodate dietary restrictions and offer delicious dishes that cater to a variety of preferences.

Whether you are a fan of street food, fusion cuisine, fermented foods, or molecular gastronomy, the Farm-to-Table movement has something to offer everyone. By supporting local farmers and producers, restaurant owners can create unique and innovative dishes that showcase the best of what the region has to offer.

In conclusion, the Farm-to-Table movement is a culinary revolution that is changing the way we think about food. By embracing this philosophy, restaurant owners, parents, families and adults can enjoy fresh, organic ingredients that are not only good for the body but also good for the planet.

Benefits of Using Fresh and Organic Ingredients

In the world of culinary arts, the use of fresh and organic ingredients has become increasingly popular among chefs and food enthusiasts alike. The benefits of incorporating these high-quality ingredients into your dishes are numerous, and they can make a significant difference in the taste, appearance, and overall quality of your food.

For restaurant owners, using fresh and organic ingredients can set your establishment apart from the competition. Customers are becoming more conscious of what they are putting into their bodies, and they appreciate restaurants that prioritize the use of high-quality, natural ingredients. By sourcing your ingredients locally and organically, you can attract a loyal customer base that values sustainability and health-conscious dining options.

Parents and adults can also benefit from incorporating fresh and organic ingredients into their daily meals. These ingredients are often more nutrient-dense and free from harmful chemicals and pesticides, making them a healthier choice for you and your family. By choosing organic produce, meats, and dairy products, you can ensure that your meals are free from harmful additives and preservatives, providing you with peace of mind about the food you are serving your loved ones.

Regardless of your dietary preferences or restrictions, fresh and organic ingredients can enhance the flavor and quality of your meals. Whether you follow a vegan, gluten-free, plant-based, or paleo diet, incorporating high-quality ingredients can help you create delicious and nutritious dishes that cater to your specific needs. From street food to fusion cuisine, farm-to-table

dining to molecular gastronomy, fresh and organic ingredients can elevate
your culinary creations and delight your taste buds.

How Farm-to-Table Dining Impacts the Restaurant Industry

Farm-to-table dining has been a growing trend in the restaurant industry in
recent years, and its impact is significant. This subchapter will explore how
this movement is changing the way restaurants operate and how it is
influencing the choices of consumers.

One of the key ways in which farm-to-table dining is impacting the restaurant
industry is by increasing the demand for locally sourced, fresh ingredients.
Restaurant owners are now more conscious of where their food comes from
and are making efforts to support local farmers and producers. This not only
benefits the local economy but also ensures that the food being served is of the
highest quality.

For parents and adults looking for healthier options, farm-to-table dining
offers a variety of fresh and organic dishes that are free from harmful
chemicals and pesticides. This makes it easier for individuals to maintain a
plant-based, paleo, or gluten-free diet. Additionally, with a focus on
sustainability and environmental consciousness, farm-to-table dining is
appealing to those who are looking to reduce their carbon footprint and
support eco-friendly practices.

Furthermore, the popularity of farm-to-table dining has led to the rise of fusion
cuisine and molecular gastronomy, where chefs are experimenting with
innovative ways to showcase local ingredients in unique and creative dishes.
This has brought a new level of excitement and creativity to the restaurant
industry, attracting food enthusiasts and adventurous eaters.

In conclusion, farm-to-table dining is not just a passing trend – it is a
movement that is here to stay. Restaurant owners who embrace this philosophy

will not only attract a wider customer base but also contribute to a more sustainable and healthy food culture.

Chapter 2: Vegan Food Creations

Vegan Appetizers

Welcome to the delicious world of vegan appetizers! Whether you are a restaurant owner looking to expand your menu, a parent wanting to introduce healthier options to your family, or just someone who loves good food, these vegan appetizers are sure to please any palate.

In the fast-paced world of restaurant dining, it can be challenging to keep up with the ever-changing demands of customers. Vegan appetizers are becoming increasingly popular as more people choose to adopt a plant-based diet. By offering a variety of vegan options on your menu, you can attract a whole new customer base and show your commitment to sustainability and health.

These vegan appetizers are not only delicious but also gluten-free and organic. Using fresh, locally sourced ingredients from the farm-to-table movement, you can create mouthwatering dishes that are as good for the planet as they are for your body. From crispy kale chips to zesty avocado hummus, there is something for everyone in these recipes.

For those looking to add a touch of fusion cuisine to their menu, try experimenting with fermented foods or molecular gastronomy techniques. Fermented vegetables can add a tangy twist to traditional appetizers, while molecular gastronomy can elevate simple ingredients to new heights of culinary creativity.

Whether you follow a plant-based diet, paleo diet, or simply love good food, these vegan appetizers are sure to satisfy your cravings. So go ahead, bring a taste of the farm-to-table movement to your table and enjoy the delicious flavors of these vegan appetizers. Your taste buds – and your customers – will thank you.

Vegan Entrees

In the world of farm-to-table dining, vegan entrees have become increasingly popular among restaurant owners and diners alike. With a focus on fresh, organic ingredients, vegan dishes offer a flavorful and nutritious option for those looking to embrace a plant-based diet.

For restaurant owners looking to expand their menu and cater to a wider audience, incorporating vegan entrees is a great way to attract customers who are seeking healthier and more sustainable dining options. By sourcing ingredients directly from local farms, restaurant owners can ensure that their vegan dishes are not only delicious but also environmentally friendly.

Parents, adults, and everyone can benefit from adding vegan entrees to their diet. Whether you are following a vegan, gluten-free, or organic diet, there are plenty of delicious options to choose from. From hearty vegetable stir-fries to creamy cashew-based pasta dishes, vegan entrees are a versatile and satisfying choice for any meal.

For those interested in exploring new culinary trends, vegan fusion cuisine offers a creative and innovative way to enjoy plant-based dishes. By combining traditional flavors and techniques with modern, innovative ingredients, restaurant owners can create unique and exciting vegan entrees that are sure to delight diners.

Whether you are a fan of fermented foods, follow a paleo diet, or are interested in molecular gastronomy, there is something for everyone to enjoy in the world of vegan entrees. With a focus on fresh, organic ingredients and innovative cooking techniques, vegan dishes offer a delicious and nutritious option for restaurant owners and diners alike.

Vegan Desserts

Vegan desserts have come a long way in recent years, proving that plant-based sweets can be just as delicious and satisfying as their traditional counterparts. In this subchapter, we will explore some creative and mouthwatering vegan dessert options that will impress your customers and leave them coming back for more.

From decadent chocolate avocado mousse to creamy coconut milk ice cream, there are endless possibilities when it comes to vegan desserts. By using fresh, organic ingredients sourced directly from local farms, you can ensure that your desserts are not only delicious but also sustainable and environmentally friendly.

For those with dietary restrictions, such as gluten-free or paleo diets, vegan desserts are a great option as they are free from animal products and often do not contain gluten or refined sugars. This makes them a versatile choice for a wide range of customers, including those with food sensitivities or allergies.

Whether you are looking to add a vegan dessert option to your menu or simply want to explore new and innovative recipes, this subchapter has something for everyone. From raw vegan cheesecake to dairy-free tiramisu, there is no shortage of delicious treats to satisfy your sweet tooth.

So why not try incorporating some vegan desserts into your restaurant's offerings and see the positive impact it can have on your customers and the environment? With farm-to-table ingredients and a creative approach to plant-based cooking, you can create desserts that are not only delicious but also ethically and sustainably sourced.

Chapter 3: Gluten-Free Delights

Understanding Gluten-Free Cooking

In recent years, gluten-free cooking has become increasingly popular among restaurant owners, parents, adults, and everyone interested in healthy eating. Gluten is a protein found in wheat, barley, and rye that can cause digestive issues for some people, particularly those with celiac disease or gluten sensitivity. By understanding gluten-free cooking, you can cater to a wider range of customers and create delicious dishes that everyone can enjoy.

When cooking gluten-free, it's important to use alternative flours such as almond flour, coconut flour, or chickpea flour in place of traditional wheat flour. These flours not only provide a gluten-free option but also add unique flavors and textures to your dishes. Additionally, it's essential to carefully read labels and avoid ingredients that may contain hidden gluten, such as soy sauce, malt vinegar, or certain seasonings.

One of the key benefits of gluten-free cooking is that it encourages the use of fresh, organic ingredients. By focusing on farm-to-table dining, you can create dishes that are not only gluten-free but also free of artificial additives and preservatives. This approach not only benefits those with gluten sensitivities but also promotes overall health and well-being for all diners.

Whether you specialize in vegan food, organic food, or fusion cuisine, understanding gluten-free cooking can help you appeal to a wider audience and showcase your creativity in the kitchen. By experimenting with different ingredients and techniques, you can create innovative dishes that are both delicious and nutritious. So why not give gluten-free cooking a try and see how it can elevate your culinary creations to new heights?

Gluten-Free Breakfast Options

In today's health-conscious world, more and more people are looking for gluten-free options when dining out. As a restaurant owner, it is essential to cater to this growing demand by offering a variety of gluten-free breakfast options on your menu. Fortunately, there are plenty of delicious and nutritious choices available that will appeal to a wide range of customers.

One popular gluten-free breakfast option is a quinoa breakfast bowl. Quinoa is a nutrient-dense grain that is naturally gluten-free and packed with protein, making it an excellent choice for those looking to start their day off right. You can top your quinoa bowl with fresh fruits, nuts, and seeds for added flavor and texture.

Another great gluten-free breakfast option is a vegetable frittata. Frittatas are easy to make and can be customized with your choice of vegetables, herbs, and cheeses. You can also add cooked bacon or sausage for a heartier option. Serve your frittata with a side of fresh fruit or a mixed green salad for a well-rounded meal.

For those with a sweet tooth, gluten-free pancakes or waffles are always a hit. You can use a gluten-free flour blend to make the batter and top your pancakes or waffles with fresh berries, maple syrup, or nut butter. You can also add chocolate chips or chopped nuts for an extra indulgent treat.

By offering a variety of gluten-free breakfast options on your menu, you can attract a wider range of customers and show that you are committed to providing fresh and organic meals for everyone. Experiment with different ingredients and flavors to create unique dishes that will keep customers coming back for more.

Gluten-Free Lunch and Dinner Recipes

Are you looking to cater to a wider range of dietary preferences at your restaurant? Look no further than our collection of gluten-free lunch and dinner recipes that are not only delicious but also easy to prepare using fresh, organic ingredients straight from the farm.

For those with gluten sensitivities or allergies, finding tasty and satisfying meals can sometimes be a challenge. That's why we've curated a selection of recipes that are not only free of gluten but also bursting with flavor and nutrients.

From hearty salads packed with seasonal vegetables to savory grain bowls featuring ancient grains like quinoa and millet, there is something for everyone in our gluten-free lunch and dinner recipes. Whether you're a vegan, following a plant-based diet, or simply looking to incorporate more organic and farm-fresh ingredients into your meals, you'll find plenty of inspiration in this chapter.

Some of our favorite gluten-free dishes include a roasted vegetable quinoa salad with a tangy lemon vinaigrette, a hearty lentil stew with root vegetables, and a creamy mushroom risotto made with arborio rice. These recipes are not only delicious but also easy to customize with your favorite herbs, spices, and proteins.

So why not impress your diners with a delicious gluten-free meal that showcases the best of farm-to-table dining? Your customers will appreciate the effort you put into creating wholesome and satisfying dishes that cater to their dietary needs. Happy cooking!

Chapter 4: Organic Kitchen Staples

Incorporating Organic Produce

In today's society, there is a growing demand for organic produce in restaurants and families kitchen. With the rise of health-conscious consumers and the desire for fresher, more sustainable options, incorporating organic ingredients into your menu can be a game-changer for your restaurant.

Organic produce is not only better for the environment, but it is also packed with nutrients and flavor. By using organic fruits and vegetables in your dishes, you are providing your customers with the highest quality ingredients that are free from harmful pesticides and chemicals.

When it comes to incorporating organic produce into your menu, the possibilities are endless. From salads and soups to entrees and desserts, there are countless ways to showcase the natural flavors of organic ingredients. Consider adding a variety of organic fruits and vegetables to your dishes, such as heirloom tomatoes, rainbow carrots, and fresh berries.

Additionally, sourcing organic produce from local farmers can help support the community and reduce your restaurant's carbon footprint. By building relationships with local farmers and suppliers, you can ensure that your ingredients are fresh, seasonal, and sustainably grown.

Whether you specialize in vegan, gluten-free, or fusion cuisine, incorporating organic produce into your menu can take your dishes to the next level. Not only will you be providing your customers with healthier options, but you will also be supporting sustainable farming practices and promoting a more environmentally friendly food system.

Overall, incorporating organic produce into your restaurant's menu is a win-win for everyone involved. From the health benefits to the delicious flavors, organic ingredients can elevate your dishes and attract a wider range of customers. So why wait? Start incorporating organic produce into your menu today and reap the benefits of fresh, flavorful, and sustainable ingredients.

Organic Meat and Poultry Dishes

Organic meat and poultry dishes are a staple in many restaurant menus, offering a delicious and sustainable option for diners looking for high-quality proteins. Whether you are a restaurant owner looking to expand your menu or a parent wanting to provide healthier meal options for your family, incorporating organic meat and poultry dishes is a great way to support local farmers and promote a more sustainable food system.

For those following a vegan or plant-based diet, there are plenty of plant-based protein options available that can be used as a substitute for meat and poultry in traditional dishes. From hearty lentil and mushroom burgers to flavorful jackfruit tacos, there are endless possibilities for creating delicious and satisfying vegan dishes that everyone will love.

If you are gluten-free or following a paleo diet, organic meat and poultry dishes are a great option as they are naturally free from gluten and processed ingredients. Try using organic chicken or grass-fed beef in stir-fries, salads, or grilled dishes for a healthy and satisfying meal that meets your dietary needs.

For those interested in fusion cuisine or molecular gastronomy, experimenting with different cooking techniques and flavor combinations can elevate traditional meat and poultry dishes to a whole new level. Try marinating organic meats in fermented sauces or incorporating unique herbs and spices to create a one-of-a-kind dining experience for your guests.

No matter your dietary preferences or culinary interests, organic meat and poultry dishes offer a delicious and sustainable option for everyone. By supporting local farmers and choosing high-quality ingredients, you can create farm-to-table feasts that are not only delicious but also good for the planet.

Using Organic Dairy Products

In the subchapter "Using Organic Dairy Products," we will explore the benefits and importance of incorporating organic dairy into your restaurant's menu. Organic dairy products come from cows that are raised without the use of antibiotics, synthetic hormones, or GMO feed. This means that the milk, cheese, and yogurt produced from these cows are free from harmful chemicals and additives, making them a healthier choice for both you and your customers.

Restaurant owners can attract health-conscious customers by offering dishes made with organic dairy products. Parents looking to provide their children with nutritious and wholesome meals will appreciate the option to choose organic dairy options on the menu. Adults who are looking to make healthier choices in their diet will also be drawn to restaurants that prioritize the use of organic ingredients.

For those following a vegan or plant-based diet, there are now a variety of plant-based alternatives to traditional dairy products such as almond milk, coconut yogurt, and cashew cheese. These options allow you to cater to a wider range of dietary preferences while still maintaining the same level of quality and flavor in your dishes.

Whether you specialize in gluten-free, street food, fusion cuisine, or molecular gastronomy, using organic dairy products can elevate the taste and quality of your dishes. From creamy risottos to rich and tangy cheesecakes, the possibilities are endless when you choose to incorporate organic dairy into your cooking.

By prioritizing the use of organic dairy products in your restaurant, you are not only supporting sustainable and ethical farming practices but also providing your customers with food that is not only delicious but also nourishing for their bodies. So go ahead, make the switch to organic dairy and reap the benefits of serving fresh and wholesome dishes to your patrons.

Chapter 5: Street Food Favorites

Popular Street Food Recipes

In this subchapter of "Farm-to-Table Feasts," we will explore some of the most popular street food recipes that are not only delicious but also fresh, organic, and perfect for restaurant owners looking to add some unique dishes to their menus. These recipes are also suitable for parents, adults, and everyone who enjoys good food, whether they follow a vegan, gluten-free, organic, or plant-based diet.

One of the most beloved street foods around the world is the classic falafel. Made from chickpeas, herbs, and spices, these crispy and flavorful little balls are perfect for a quick and satisfying meal. Serve them in pita bread with some fresh veggies and tahini sauce for an authentic experience.

For those looking for a gluten-free option, try making Vietnamese summer rolls. These light and refreshing rolls are filled with fresh vegetables, herbs, and either shrimp or tofu, making them a healthy and delicious choice for a light lunch or snack.

If you're a fan of fusion cuisine, why not try making Korean BBQ tacos? Fill soft corn tortillas with marinated and grilled meat or tofu, kimchi, and a spicy sauce for a unique and flavorful twist on traditional street food.

No matter what type of cuisine you prefer, there is something for everyone in the world of street food. So whether you're a fan of fermented foods, follow a paleo diet, or are interested in molecular gastronomy, these popular street food recipes are sure to satisfy your cravings and impress your customers.

Putting a Gourmet Twist on Street Food

In recent years, street food has gained a reputation as being quick, affordable, and delicious. But what if we told you that you could elevate this humble cuisine to gourmet status? In this subchapter, we will explore how restaurant owners can put a gourmet twist on street food, catering to a variety of dietary preferences and tastes.

One way to elevate street food is by incorporating fresh, organic ingredients sourced directly from local farms. By embracing the farm-to-table philosophy, restaurant owners can ensure that their dishes are not only delicious but also sustainable and environmentally friendly. Whether you're serving up vegan tacos or gluten-free burgers, using organic produce and ethically raised meats can take your street food offerings to the next level.

For those looking to add a unique twist to their street food menu, fusion cuisine is the way to go. By combining different culinary traditions and flavors, restaurant owners can create innovative dishes that will keep customers coming back for more. Imagine Korean BBQ tacos, Thai-inspired noodle bowls, or Mexican-style sushi rolls – the possibilities are endless!

If you're catering to health-conscious customers, consider offering fermented foods or plant-based options on your street food menu. Fermented foods like kimchi and sauerkraut are not only delicious but also packed with probiotics and other gut-friendly nutrients. Plant-based dishes, on the other hand, are a great way to cater to vegans and vegetarians while still offering mouth-watering options for all diners.

In conclusion, putting a gourmet twist on street food is a great way to attract customers and set your restaurant apart from the competition. Whether you're serving up vegan, gluten-free, or organic dishes, there are plenty of ways to elevate your street food offerings and create a dining experience that will keep customers coming back for more.

Street Food Inspired Desserts

Are you looking to add a unique and delicious twist to your dessert menu? Look no further than street food inspired desserts! Drawing inspiration from the vibrant and diverse world of street food, these desserts offer a fun and innovative take on traditional sweet treats.

Whether you're a restaurant owner looking to spice up your menu, a parent searching for new and exciting recipes to try at home, or an adult with a sweet tooth, street food inspired desserts are sure to delight your taste buds. With influences from around the globe, these desserts combine bold flavors and unexpected ingredients to create a truly memorable dining experience.

From vegan churros drizzled with dairy-free chocolate sauce to gluten-free mochi ice cream, there's something for everyone to enjoy. For those following a plant-based diet, try a refreshing coconut mango sticky rice, or indulge in a decadent avocado chocolate mousse for a healthy yet satisfying treat.

If you're a fan of fusion cuisine, experiment with flavors and textures by combining traditional street food ingredients with classic dessert recipes. Think savory-sweet miso caramel popcorn or spicy chili-infused chocolate truffles for a culinary adventure unlike any other.

Whether you're a fan of organic, gluten-free, or vegan food, street food inspired desserts offer a creative and delicious way to satisfy your sweet tooth. So why not take a culinary journey around the world with these innovative and mouthwatering dessert recipes? Your taste buds will thank you!

Chapter 6: Fusion Cuisine Experiments

Fusion Cuisine Basics

In the world of culinary arts, fusion cuisine has become increasingly popular for its innovative and exciting blend of flavors from different cultures. In this subchapter, we will explore the basics of fusion cuisine and how you can incorporate it into your restaurant's menu.

Fusion cuisine is all about mixing and matching ingredients and cooking techniques from various culinary traditions to create unique and delicious dishes. The key to successful fusion cuisine is to balance the flavors and textures of the different ingredients to create a harmonious dish that is greater than the sum of its parts.

When creating fusion dishes, it is important to start with high-quality, fresh ingredients. This is where farm-to-table dining becomes essential. By sourcing your ingredients from local farms and producers, you can ensure that your dishes are not only delicious but also sustainable and environmentally friendly.

For those with dietary restrictions or preferences, fusion cuisine can also be adapted to accommodate vegan, gluten-free, and organic diets. By using plant-based ingredients, gluten-free grains, and organic produce, you can create fusion dishes that are not only delicious but also healthy and nutritious.

Experimenting with fermented foods, such as kimchi or sauerkraut, can add a unique depth of flavor to your fusion dishes. Similarly, incorporating elements of molecular gastronomy, such as foams or gels, can elevate your dishes to a whole new level of creativity and sophistication.

Whether you are a restaurant owner looking to revamp your menu or a home cook looking to impress your family and friends, fusion cuisine is a versatile and exciting culinary trend that is sure to delight your taste buds. So go ahead, experiment with different flavors and ingredients, and let your creativity shine through in your fusion dishes.

Asian Fusion Recipes

In recent years, Asian fusion cuisine has become increasingly popular in the culinary world. This innovative style of cooking combines traditional Asian ingredients and cooking techniques with flavors and ingredients from other cuisines. The result is a delicious and unique blend of flavors that will tantalize your taste buds.

For restaurant owners looking to add some excitement to their menus, incorporating Asian fusion recipes can be a great way to attract new customers and keep existing ones coming back for more. Whether you're looking to offer vegan, gluten-free, or organic options, there are plenty of Asian fusion recipes that can be tailored to meet the needs of your diners.

From savory stir-fries to spicy curries, there are endless possibilities when it comes to creating Asian fusion dishes. Try incorporating ingredients like tofu, tempeh, and a variety of fresh vegetables to create healthy and delicious meals that everyone will love. For those following a plant-based or paleo diet, there are plenty of options that can be easily adapted to meet your dietary restrictions.

For parents looking to introduce their children to new and exciting flavors, Asian fusion recipes can be a great way to expand their palates and encourage them to try new foods. From crispy spring rolls to flavorful noodle dishes, there are plenty of kid-friendly options that are sure to please even the pickiest eaters.

No matter what your dietary preferences may be, there is something for everyone to enjoy when it comes to Asian fusion recipes. So why not spice up your menu with some delicious and innovative dishes that will have your customers coming back for more?

Mediterranean Fusion Dishes

In this subchapter on Mediterranean Fusion Dishes, we explore the diverse and delicious flavors of the Mediterranean region combined with innovative fusion techniques. Restaurant owners looking to offer unique and exciting dishes on their menus will find inspiration in these fresh and organic recipes.

For parents and adults seeking healthy and flavorful meal options, Mediterranean fusion dishes are a great choice. These dishes often incorporate a variety of fresh vegetables, legumes, whole grains, and lean proteins, making them a nutritious and satisfying choice for any meal.

For those following a vegan, gluten-free, or organic diet, Mediterranean fusion dishes offer plenty of options. From vibrant salads and hearty grain bowls to flavorful wraps and tasty mezze platters, there is something for everyone in this chapter.

Fans of street food will love the bold and vibrant flavors of Mediterranean fusion dishes. Whether it's a falafel wrap with harissa aioli or a grilled vegetable skewer with tzatziki sauce, these dishes are sure to please any palate.

For those interested in fusion cuisine, Mediterranean fusion dishes offer a unique blend of traditional Mediterranean flavors with modern cooking techniques. From deconstructed moussaka to smoked eggplant hummus, these dishes are sure to impress even the most discerning foodies.

Whether you are a fan of farm-to-table dining, fermented foods, plant-based or paleo diets, or molecular gastronomy, there is something for everyone in this subchapter on Mediterranean Fusion Dishes. Get ready to tantalize your taste buds with these creative and delicious recipes that celebrate the best of Mediterranean cuisine.

Chapter 7: Fermented Foods for Flavor

Introduction to Fermentation

In the world of farm-to-table dining, fermentation plays a vital role in creating unique and flavorful dishes. From tangy kimchi to tangy kombucha, fermented foods are not only delicious but also packed with health benefits. In this subchapter, we will explore the fascinating process of fermentation and how it can be incorporated into your restaurant's menu.

Fermentation is a natural process where microorganisms, such as bacteria, yeast, and molds, break down sugars and starches in food, creating compounds like alcohol and organic acids. This process not only preserves food but also enhances its flavor and nutritional value. Fermented foods are rich in probiotics, which promote gut health and boost the immune system.

For restaurant owners looking to add fermented foods to their menu, there are endless possibilities. From pickles and sauerkraut to miso and tempeh, fermented foods can be incorporated into a variety of dishes, adding depth and complexity to flavors. For parents looking to introduce their children to new and exciting foods, fermented foods are a great way to expand their palates and introduce them to different cultures.

Adults looking to improve their health and well-being can benefit from incorporating fermented foods into their diet. Whether following a vegan, gluten-free, organic, or plant-based diet, fermented foods are a versatile and delicious addition to any meal. For those following a paleo or molecular gastronomy diet, fermented foods can add a unique twist to traditional dishes.

In this subchapter, we will explore the many benefits of fermentation and provide recipes and tips for incorporating fermented foods into your restaurant's menu. Whether you are a seasoned chef or a home cook, fermentation is a simple and rewarding process that can elevate your dishes to new heights. So join us on this culinary journey and discover the magic of fermentation.

Fermented Vegetable Recipes

Fermented vegetables are a staple in many traditional diets around the world, and for good reason. Not only do they add a unique tangy flavor to dishes, but they are also packed with probiotics and other beneficial nutrients that support gut health and overall well-being. In this subchapter, we will explore some delicious and creative fermented vegetable recipes that you can incorporate into your restaurant menu or make at home.

One popular fermented vegetable dish is kimchi, a Korean staple made with cabbage, radishes, and a spicy chili paste. This tangy and spicy condiment is perfect for adding a kick to rice bowls, tacos, or even stir-fries. Another classic fermented vegetable recipe is sauerkraut, which is made with cabbage and salt and can be used as a topping for hot dogs, sandwiches, or salads.

For those looking for a more exotic twist, consider experimenting with fermented vegetables from other cultures. For example, you can try making curtido, a Salvadoran fermented cabbage slaw that pairs perfectly with pupusas or grilled meats. Or, venture into the world of Japanese cuisine with tsukemono, a variety of pickled vegetables that are often served as a side dish or snack.

Whether you are a fan of vegan, gluten-free, or organic food, fermented vegetables are a versatile and delicious addition to any diet. By incorporating these recipes into your menu, you can offer your customers a unique and healthy dining experience that they won't soon forget. So roll up your sleeves, grab your mason jars, and start fermenting your way to a healthier and more flavorful menu.

Fermented Drink Ideas

In this subchapter, we will explore the world of fermented drink ideas that are not only delicious but also packed with probiotics and nutrients. Fermented drinks have been gaining popularity in recent years for their health benefits and unique flavors. From kombucha to kefir, there are so many options to choose from when it comes to incorporating fermented drinks into your menu.

One popular fermented drink that you may want to consider adding to your restaurant menu is kombucha. Kombucha is a fizzy, tangy drink made from fermented tea that is rich in probiotics and antioxidants. It comes in a variety of flavors, making it a versatile option for any type of cuisine. You can even experiment with different fruit and herb infusions to create your own signature kombucha flavors.

Another fermented drink idea to consider is water kefir. Water kefir is a dairy-free alternative to traditional kefir that is made from fermented sugar water. It has a slightly sweet and tangy flavor, making it a refreshing beverage option for those looking for a non-alcoholic alternative. You can serve water kefir plain or add in different fruit juices for a burst of flavor.

For those looking for a more traditional fermented drink option, consider offering homemade ginger beer. Ginger beer is a spicy and slightly sweet drink made from fermented ginger, sugar, and water. It is a great option for those looking for a non-alcoholic beverage with a kick.

Overall, incorporating fermented drinks into your menu can be a great way to offer your customers unique and healthy beverage options. Whether you are looking to appeal to the vegan, gluten-free, or organic food niches, fermented drinks are a versatile and delicious addition to any restaurant menu. Cheers to good health and great flavors!

Chapter 8: Plant-Based Diet Options

Building a Plant-Based Menu

In today's culinary landscape, plant-based menus are becoming increasingly popular among restaurant owners, parents, adults, and everyone in between. Whether you are catering to vegan, gluten-free, organic, or health-conscious customers, incorporating plant-based dishes into your menu can attract a wider audience and showcase your commitment to fresh and sustainable ingredients.

When building a plant-based menu, it is important to focus on creativity, flavor, and nutritional balance. Incorporating a variety of fruits, vegetables, grains, legumes, nuts, and seeds can provide a diverse range of nutrients and flavors that will appeal to a broad spectrum of tastes.

Consider offering plant-based versions of classic dishes, such as vegan burgers, plant-based tacos, or gluten-free pasta dishes. Experiment with different cooking techniques and flavor profiles to create unique and exciting plant-based options that will keep customers coming back for more.

Incorporating fermented foods, such as kimchi, sauerkraut, or kombucha, can add depth and complexity to plant-based dishes while also promoting gut health. Additionally, exploring fusion cuisine and molecular gastronomy techniques can take your plant-based menu to the next level, offering innovative and visually stunning dishes that will impress even the most discerning diners.

Whether you are following a plant-based diet, paleo diet, or simply looking to incorporate more plant-based options into your menu, building a plant-based menu can be a rewarding and delicious endeavor. By sourcing fresh, organic ingredients from local farms and producers, you can create a farm-to-table dining experience that highlights the beauty and flavor of plant-based cuisine.

Plant-Based Breakfast Ideas

For restaurant owners looking to cater to the growing demand for plant-based options, breakfast can be a great place to start. Plant-based breakfast ideas not only appeal to vegans and vegetarians, but also to health-conscious individuals looking to start their day with a nutritious meal.

One popular plant-based breakfast idea is a smoothie bowl. These bowls typically consist of a blend of fruits, vegetables, and plant-based milk or yogurt topped with granola, nuts, seeds, and other toppings. They are not only delicious, but also visually appealing and can be customized to suit different tastes.

Another plant-based breakfast option is avocado toast. This simple yet satisfying dish consists of mashed avocado spread on whole grain toast, topped with ingredients like cherry tomatoes, arugula, and a drizzle of balsamic glaze. Avocado toast is a great way to showcase fresh, organic ingredients in a flavorful and filling dish.

For those looking for a heartier breakfast option, a tofu scramble can be a great choice. Tofu, when seasoned and cooked with vegetables like bell peppers, onions, and spinach, can mimic the taste and texture of scrambled eggs. Tofu scrambles can be served with a side of roasted potatoes or whole grain toast for a satisfying and protein-packed meal.

By incorporating these plant-based breakfast ideas into their menus, restaurant owners can attract a wider range of customers and showcase their commitment to fresh, organic, and sustainable ingredients. Whether for vegans, vegetarians, or those simply looking to add more plant-based options to their diet, these breakfast ideas are sure to please a diverse range of palates.

Plant-Based Dinner Creations

In today's culinary landscape, plant-based dining is becoming increasingly popular among consumers looking for healthier and more sustainable options. Restaurant owners can capitalize on this trend by offering innovative and delicious plant-based dinner creations that cater to a wide range of dietary preferences and restrictions.

For parents looking to introduce more plant-based meals into their family's diet, these recipes offer a perfect opportunity to get creative in the kitchen. With options ranging from hearty grain bowls to flavorful vegetable stir-fries, there is something for everyone to enjoy.

Adults looking to explore new flavors and ingredients will also be delighted by the diverse range of plant-based dinner creations included in this subchapter. From vibrant salads to comforting soups and stews, these recipes showcase the versatility and deliciousness of plant-based cuisine.

For those following a vegan, gluten-free, or organic diet, these recipes provide a wealth of options that are both nutritious and satisfying. With a focus on fresh, seasonal ingredients sourced from local farms, these dishes highlight the beauty and flavor of plant-based cooking.

Restaurant owners looking to expand their menu offerings can find inspiration in these plant-based dinner creations. Whether incorporating elements of street food, fusion cuisine, or molecular gastronomy, there are endless possibilities for creating innovative and exciting plant-based dishes that will appeal to a wide range of diners.

Incorporating fermented foods, farm-to-table ingredients, and Paleo-friendly options, these recipes offer a comprehensive guide to creating plant-based dinners that are both delicious and nutritious. Whether you are a seasoned chef or a home cook looking to explore new culinary horizons, these plant-based dinner creations are sure to inspire and delight.

Chapter 9: Paleo Diet Innovations

Paleo Diet Principles

The Paleo diet, also known as the caveman diet, is based on the idea of eating foods that our ancestors would have consumed during the Paleolithic era. This means focusing on whole, unprocessed foods such as lean meats, fish, fruits, vegetables, nuts, and seeds. The Paleo diet excludes grains, dairy, and processed foods, as these were not available to our ancestors.

One of the key principles of the Paleo diet is to prioritize high-quality, organic ingredients. By choosing organic produce, grass-fed meats, and wild-caught fish, you can ensure that you are getting the most nutrient-dense foods possible. This not only benefits your health but also supports sustainable farming practices.

Another important principle of the Paleo diet is to avoid processed sugars and artificial ingredients. Instead, focus on natural sweeteners like honey or maple syrup, and use herbs and spices to add flavor to your dishes. By cutting out processed foods, you can reduce inflammation in the body and improve overall health.

For restaurant owners looking to incorporate Paleo principles into their menu, consider offering grass-fed burgers, roasted vegetables, and salads with homemade dressings. You can also experiment with Paleo-friendly desserts using almond flour and coconut sugar.

Parents and adults can also benefit from following Paleo principles in their own home cooking. By focusing on whole, unprocessed foods, you can support your overall health and well-being. Whether you are looking to lose weight, improve digestion, or increase energy levels, the Paleo diet can be a great option for everyone.

In conclusion, the Paleo diet emphasizes the importance of eating whole, unprocessed foods that our ancestors would have consumed. By following these principles, you can support your health, the environment, and local farmers. Consider incorporating Paleo principles into your own cooking and dining experiences for a truly farm-to-table feast.

Paleo-Friendly Snacks

In the world of restaurant dining, catering to different dietary preferences and restrictions has become increasingly important. One popular diet that has gained traction in recent years is the Paleo diet, which focuses on consuming whole foods that our ancestors would have eaten. For restaurant owners looking to appeal to Paleo enthusiasts, offering Paleo-friendly snacks is a great way to attract this niche market.

Paleo-friendly snacks are not only delicious, but they are also made with fresh, organic ingredients that adhere to the principles of the Paleo diet. These snacks are free from grains, dairy, and processed sugars, making them a healthier alternative to traditional snack options. Restaurant owners can easily incorporate Paleo-friendly snacks into their menu by offering items such as nut and seed bars, vegetable chips, and coconut-based treats.

Parents looking for nutritious snacks for their children will appreciate the variety of options available on the menu. Adults following a Paleo diet will also find these snacks to be a satisfying and guilt-free indulgence. Everyone can benefit from the wholesome ingredients and delicious flavors that Paleo-friendly snacks have to offer.

By including Paleo-friendly snacks on the menu, restaurant owners can attract a wider range of customers, including those with vegan, gluten-free, and organic dietary preferences. These snacks can also be incorporated into street food and fusion cuisine offerings, making them a versatile option for any type of restaurant. Whether you specialize in farm-to-table dining, fermented foods, plant-based cuisine, or molecular gastronomy, Paleo-friendly snacks are a great addition to your menu.

Paleo Dessert Recipes

In this subchapter on Paleo dessert recipes, we will explore delicious and nutritious treats that are free from grains, refined sugars, and processed ingredients. These recipes are perfect for those following a Paleo diet, as well as anyone looking for healthier dessert options.

One of the most popular Paleo dessert recipes is a coconut flour chocolate cake. This moist and decadent cake is made with coconut flour, coconut oil, raw honey, and dark chocolate. It is rich in flavor and has a fudgy texture that will satisfy your sweet tooth without any guilt.

For a lighter option, try making Paleo-friendly fruit sorbet. This refreshing dessert is made with frozen fruit, coconut milk, and a touch of honey or maple syrup. It is a great way to cool off on a hot summer day while still sticking to your Paleo diet.

If you are a fan of cookies, you will love our almond butter cookies recipe. These chewy and nutty cookies are made with almond butter, coconut sugar, and a hint of vanilla. They are a great snack or dessert option for those following a Paleo diet.

No Paleo dessert recipe collection would be complete without a recipe for avocado chocolate mousse. This creamy and indulgent dessert is made with ripe avocados, cocoa powder, and a touch of honey. It is a great way to sneak some healthy fats into your diet while satisfying your chocolate cravings.

These Paleo dessert recipes are not only delicious but also easy to make. They are perfect for restaurant owners looking to expand their menu with healthier options, as well as parents and adults looking to incorporate more Paleo-friendly treats into their diet. Give these recipes a try and indulge in guilt-free desserts that are sure to impress your taste buds.

Chapter 10: Exploring Molecular Gastronomy

Molecular Gastronomy Techniques

Molecular gastronomy techniques have revolutionized the way we think about food preparation and presentation. By utilizing scientific principles and cutting-edge technology, chefs can create dishes that are not only visually stunning but also bursting with unique flavors and textures.

One of the most popular molecular gastronomy techniques is spherification, which involves turning liquids into small spheres that burst in your mouth. This technique is perfect for adding a touch of whimsy to your dishes and can be used to create everything from flavorful caviar-like beads to fruit-filled spheres.

Another popular technique is foams, which are created by using a siphon to aerate liquids. Foams are a great way to add a light and airy texture to your dishes, and can be flavored with a variety of ingredients such as herbs, spices, or fruits.

Gelification is another common technique in molecular gastronomy, which involves turning liquids into gels using gelling agents such as agar or gelatin. This technique is perfect for creating dishes with unique textures, such as creamy gels or firm jellies.

Overall, molecular gastronomy techniques offer endless possibilities for creativity in the kitchen. By incorporating these techniques into your cooking repertoire, you can elevate your dishes to new heights and impress your customers with innovative and delicious creations. So why not experiment with spherification, foams, and gelification in your restaurant today? Your taste buds will thank you!

Molecular Gastronomy Appetizers

Molecular gastronomy has become a popular trend in the culinary world, offering a unique and innovative approach to cooking. In this subchapter, we will explore how restaurant owners can incorporate molecular gastronomy techniques into their appetizer menus to create exciting and memorable dishes for their customers.

One of the key principles of molecular gastronomy is the use of scientific techniques to transform familiar ingredients into unexpected textures and flavors. By utilizing tools such as spherification, emulsification, and foaming, chefs can create appetizers that are not only visually stunning but also incredibly delicious.

For vegan and gluten-free options, restaurant owners can experiment with ingredients such as agar agar, xanthan gum, and aquafaba to create plant-based versions of classic appetizers. Imagine serving a vegan "caviar" made from seaweed extract or a gluten-free "foam" made from chickpea brine – these dishes are sure to impress even the most discerning diners.

For those interested in organic and farm-to-table dining, molecular gastronomy offers endless possibilities for showcasing the natural flavors of fresh, locally sourced ingredients. Consider serving a deconstructed caprese salad with mozzarella spheres and tomato foam, or a modern take on bruschetta with balsamic pearls and basil air.

Whether you are catering to a plant-based, paleo, or fusion cuisine crowd, molecular gastronomy can elevate your appetizer menu to new heights. By experimenting with innovative techniques and ingredients, restaurant owners can create dishes that are not only delicious but also a feast for the eyes. So go ahead, embrace the world of molecular gastronomy and watch as your customers delight in the culinary magic you have created.

Molecular Gastronomy Desserts

Welcome to the exciting world of Molecular Gastronomy Desserts! In this subchapter, we will explore how you can incorporate cutting-edge culinary techniques into your restaurant's dessert menu to create innovative and unforgettable dishes that will delight your customers.

Molecular Gastronomy is a culinary movement that combines science and art to create dishes that not only taste amazing but also have a visually stunning presentation. By using techniques such as spherification, foams, gels, and emulsions, you can elevate your desserts to a whole new level.

For restaurant owners looking to cater to a diverse range of dietary preferences and restrictions, Molecular Gastronomy Desserts offer a wealth of possibilities. Whether your customers are vegan, gluten-free, or following a plant-based or paleo diet, you can create desserts that are not only delicious but also meet their specific needs.

Parents will also appreciate the creativity and innovation that Molecular Gastronomy Desserts bring to the table. By offering desserts that are both fun and nutritious, you can encourage children to explore new flavors and textures while also providing them with a healthy treat.

Adults of all ages will be impressed by the unique flavors and textures of Molecular Gastronomy Desserts. Whether they are looking for a sweet indulgence or a sophisticated dessert option, these dishes are sure to please even the most discerning palates.

So why not take your dessert menu to the next level with Molecular Gastronomy? With a little creativity and experimentation, you can create desserts that are not only delicious and visually stunning but also cater to a wide range of dietary preferences and restrictions. Your customers will thank you for it!

Chapter 11: Conclusion and Next Steps

Tips for Implementing Farm-to-Table Practices in Your Restaurant

Implementing farm-to-table practices in your restaurant can be a rewarding experience for both you and your customers. By using fresh, locally sourced ingredients, you can create dishes that are not only delicious but also sustainable and environmentally friendly. Here are some tips to help you successfully incorporate farm-to-table practices into your restaurant:

1. Build relationships with local farmers and suppliers: Get to know the people who grow your food and develop strong partnerships with them. This will not only ensure that you have a steady supply of fresh ingredients, but it will also help support your local community.

2. Update your menu regularly: One of the benefits of using local, seasonal ingredients is that your menu can change frequently to reflect what is available. Embrace this flexibility and update your menu regularly to showcase the freshest ingredients.

3. Educate your staff and customers: Make sure your staff is knowledgeable about where your ingredients come from and the benefits of using locally sourced produce. Educate your customers as well by highlighting the farm-to-table practices in your restaurant and the importance of supporting local farmers.

4. Be creative with your dishes: Experiment with different flavor combinations and cooking techniques to make the most of your fresh ingredients. Get creative with your menu items to showcase the quality of the produce you are using.

5. Embrace sustainability: In addition to sourcing local ingredients, consider other sustainable practices such as composting food waste, using eco-friendly packaging, and reducing water and energy consumption in your restaurant.

By following these tips, you can successfully implement farm-to-table practices in your restaurant and provide your customers with fresh, delicious, and sustainable meals. Your efforts will not only benefit your business but also support local farmers and promote a healthier, more environmentally friendly food system.

Planning Your Farm-to-Table Menu

In the world of farm-to-table dining, planning your menu is essential to creating a successful and sustainable restaurant. Whether you are a seasoned restaurant owner or just starting out, understanding how to create a menu that highlights fresh, organic ingredients is key.

When planning your farm-to-table menu, it's important to consider the seasonality of ingredients. By using locally sourced produce that is in season, you can ensure that your dishes are not only delicious but also environmentally friendly. This also allows you to support local farmers and create a stronger connection with your community.

Another important factor to consider when planning your farm-to-table menu is dietary restrictions. With the rise in popularity of vegan, gluten-free, and organic diets, it's important to offer a variety of options for your customers. By including dishes that cater to these dietary restrictions, you can attract a wider range of customers and ensure that everyone has something delicious to enjoy.

For those looking to add a unique twist to their farm-to-table menu, consider incorporating elements of street food, fusion cuisine, or fermented foods. These culinary trends can add a fun and adventurous element to your menu, while still highlighting the fresh and organic ingredients that are the foundation of farm-to-table dining.

Whether you follow a plant-based, paleo, or molecular gastronomy diet, there are endless possibilities when it comes to planning your farm-to-table menu. By taking the time to carefully consider seasonality, dietary restrictions, and culinary trends, you can create a menu that is not only delicious but also sustainable and environmentally friendly. So get creative, experiment with new ingredients, and let your farm-to-table menu shine!

Resources for Finding Fresh and Organic Ingredients

In order to create delicious farm-to-table feasts using fresh and organic ingredients, it is crucial to know where to find the best products. Luckily, there are numerous resources available for restaurant owners, parents, adults, and everyone else interested in cooking with high-quality ingredients.

For those looking to source fresh produce, either for agro businesses, restocking, agro-business distribution, local farmers markets are a great place to start. These markets often feature a wide variety of fruits, vegetables, seeds, grains, roots, cereals and herbs that are grown locally and sustainably. By purchasing from farmers markets, you can support small-scale farmers and ensure that your ingredients are as fresh as possible.

Another excellent resource for finding fresh and organic ingredients is community-supported agriculture (CSA) programs. Through a CSA, individuals can purchase a share of a local farm's harvest and receive a weekly delivery of seasonal produce. This is a fantastic way to get a regular supply of fresh ingredients while supporting small-scale agriculture in your community.

For those looking for specialty ingredients such as organic grains, spices, or fermented foods, online retailers like Thrive Market or specialty health food stores are great options. These retailers often carry a wide selection of organic and specialty products that can elevate your dishes to the next level.

Additionally, for those interested in molecular gastronomy or fusion cuisine, there are specialized suppliers that offer unique ingredients like agar agar, liquid nitrogen, or exotic spices. These suppliers can help you create cutting-edge dishes that will impress even the most discerning diners.

No matter what type of cuisine you specialize in, there are resources available to help you find the freshest and most organic ingredients for your farm-to-table feasts. By sourcing high-quality ingredients, you can create dishes that are not only delicious but also environmentally sustainable and socially responsible.